I MIGHT BE
SCHIZOPHRENIC,
BUT I'M NOT
CRAZY

FRANCINE FUENTES

Paperback ISBN: 978-1-63616-012-2

Published by Opportune Independent Publishing Company

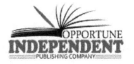

For permission requests, write to the publisher, addressed "Attention: Permissions Coordinator" to the address below.

Email: Info@opportunepublishing.com

Address: 113 N. Live Oak Street
Houston, TX 77003

For more information, and to contact Francine Fuentes, please visit www.FrancineFuentes.com

"This book of poetry is a much needed wake-up call about living with a psychotic disorder that takes an incredible amount of work. Francine knows that having a family member with this mental illness on medication still will experience symptoms which can onerous and intrusive. Francine writes from the heart and her experiences."

—Joseph A. Laguna, M.D.

"Francine Fuentes writes a remarkable book of short poems about her family which includes a brother with mental illness, Schizophrenia. Trying to survive in a family where the effects of mental illness takes its toll on everyone in different ways. Fran often finds herself as the sole caretaker of her brother, trying to please her parents but often losing her own identity. A very emotional journey trying to hold on and not fall in the darkness below, struggling to love and find her own way and meaning in her own life, yet never letting go of her love and care of her brother."

—Irv Hoffman, Mental Health Counselor

"Mental illness creates barriers for so many. For far too long, it was not understood, and victims of mental illness were viewed as inferior. Luckily, as society continues to come to grips with the reality that anyone could be impacted, we can start to see beyond someone's mental illness and instead glimpse into their humanity. Through her poetry and reflections, Francine Fuentes gives us a glimpse of the beauty and trauma that comes with growing up and caring for a brother with schizophrenia, and how that transformed her outlook on life – both positively and negatively. Her poems and stories are empowering to anyone who feels alone in their struggles, and takes the reader through a variety of experiences and emotions."

—Chris Lumia, Ed.S.

"Francine has found a refreshingly imaginative way to share her experiences with mental illness through beautiful poetry. It's truly a unique, thought provoking and educational perspective."

—Christine Tripp
Director of Student Recruitment and Enrollment
Marketing Services at Eastern Florida State College

"Francine's book of poetry is very well done. The moment I started to read through the poems I could feel the pressure and pain of her life as she grew. She brings to light the challenges of loving and taking care of a person with special needs, particularly schizophrenia. These poems clearly show the unpredictable implications this disorder can have on a person. Though the majority of the poems in this book are short, they are equally powerful and will speak to anyone with a difficult past and/or experience in dealing first hand with a loved one who suffers from unpredictability of a mental illness. This book is also motivational and clearly shows that anyone can succeed in life despite their past experiences and where they have been. Francine confirms that a little kindness and understanding can go a long way toward achieving success in life. I highly recommend this wonderful read for anyone who needs to know that there are others out there that share a similar experience both of a troubling past and of how it feels to love someone who can be emotionally unstable."

—Amy S. English, MS
Student Success Advisor II and Professor of History and
Student Life Skills at Florida SouthWestern State College

Grateful To

My brother whose strength amazes me. You are the reason! You are the hero! You are brilliant! You are loved!

My husband, Al, our son Gabriel and Maya for believing in me.

Family! My parents. Your job was difficult. Mine was too! I have become stronger, self-sufficient and a loving parent. I learned I have unlimited potential.

My gracious neighbor who introduced me to my mentor who wishes to remain anonymous.

My cousin, Lisa Ozalis-Graham for the push with love! And, to Stan Ozalis and family for helping my brother in too many ways to mention.

My friend Lynn Brooks who reminded me to keep it real!

To the man that brought food to my brother and kept me abreast of his needs.

Finally, I am eternally grateful to all who treat my brother kindly ***when no one is watching.***

Introduction

Writing this book has been a journey unlike any I have experienced. Family shapes the first years of our lives. Our upbringing is critical to the type of people we may become when we reach adulthood. When a family member is mentally ill, the entire structure often breaks down. Children become the parents and feel emotionally responsible for their wellbeing. The parents become children. The weight is heavy! Protecting my brother who is afflicted with paranoid schizophrenia became my job. My mom and dad didn't know what to do, nor did I, his older sister who was parentified before entering the second grade.

No matter what, a dysfunctional family will affect most of its members to the point that it can cause mental illness, depression and trauma such as PTSD.

I kept my distance for a number of years because I didn't think my brother wanted me to visit and I was full of anxiety. We then reconnected. I'm grateful for whatever time we have together. The climate of our visits vary. Some are the way I envision and others are just what they are. There is no rhyme or reason.

This could apply to other families. I hope that when you see someone that looks, acts or speaks differently than you, that you will remember they are someone's child. Take a moment to smile, listen or perhaps offer a meal or some change.

Their hell is forever. Your joy could be in the moment of just being there for another human being. To quote the late Carrie Fisher "Turn your broken heart into Art."

This is my truth.
BE THE DIFFERENCE!

Chapter 1: My Brother

I AM Schizophrenic but I'm NOT crazy

"There will be a cure someday but I don't think I will be here to see it."

My brother

FEAR

I'm scared
They're chasing me
It reminds me of when
I was committed
But you begin to feel better again
Right?
Yes, the feeling goes away
But it always returns
With all it's might!
Just another day

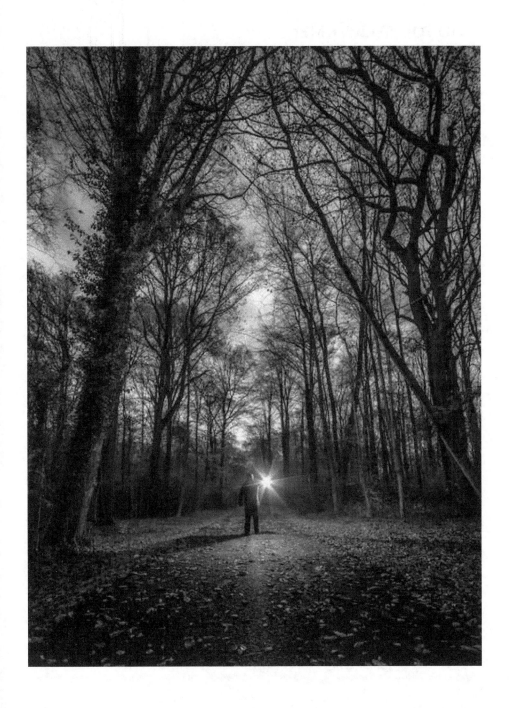

DO YOU BELIEVE ME?

They did things to me!
Do you believe me?
They came into my room at night
I had no rights!
They drugged me
Til I had no fight
Tell me you believe me!

BUDDY

Your Buddy
Friend, companion
Throughout the strife
You fed, cuddled
So much love
You slept together
You were one
True blue
Visits to the Vet
And yet, you were poor
You put him first
To be sure he was satisfied
With food and thirst
A Basic need
Then Buddy could rest
The sweet boy Buddy
Innocence indeed
But sometimes the
Voices would upset you
And suffering
Began
Alone with
You
The secrets, depression, sickness
Appeared
The secrets with Buddy
Went to his grave
Your connection never ceased
Look up to the sky, says Buddy
And feel the breeze
A life of sunshine, peace and soft caresses
I loved you my master
You were my life
I look down and remember your hell
And pray in dog heaven
That you will be well

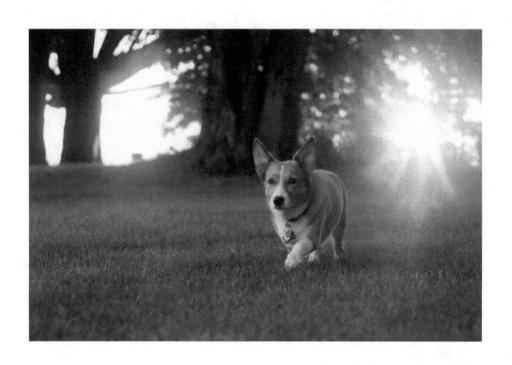

OUR NEIGHBOR

You reminded me that our neighbor
Was always there for you
She bought you clothes
Gave you money
Always kind
Our neighbor has passed
It's nice that you have a few
Good memories and that our neighbor
Showered you with kindness

WRITER

I can no longer write
My thoughts on paper
My meds prevent my
Thoughts to be shared

My hand doesn't work
Using a pen
I have so much to say
That needs to be heard
Will you share them?

FOOD STAMPS

You have food stamps
No energy to shop
Climbing the stairs
To your home
Is a major task
Hard for you to breathe
No Strength
For the food you need

THE MAZE

Each day
I travel by foot
Returning to the same place
Turns, corners
Paths I create
Lead to no options
I'm smart
I know I am
Push the webs away!
Open my world!

THEY ARE WATCHING ME

They're ready to take me
From outside my door
It's true!
I don't know what to do
If they get me
I won't return
Cops or something
In between
They'll take my life
I can't scream
Inside my arm
They'll insert
Some sort of gadget
That draws my blood
Until my brain melts down
They'll tell
Their people
 To watch me
They always do
I need help please
They won't hurt you – it's not real
You don't believe me
But it's true
Is your mind playing tricks on you?

CIGARETTES

The cup by your door
Houses ashes
That endure
Each and every day
The container is
Filled with
Butts by the dozen
You surround it with you
Each day it grew
Coke in the glass
Hold the remains
Of smoke you inhale
Your breathing
In pain

MOMMY AND DADDY

You wish they were here
You cry for them now
They loved you so much
You seemed to lose trust
They could never be in your place
As no one can
We hurt for you always
They prayed for a plan
To bring hope and a cure
In your lifetime indeed
To rid of the voices
You hear
Every day
That God will take your heart
And shoot it with faith
You continue to be loved
And I promise you won't leave without a trace

TELEPHONE RINGS

The phone call
Hello my brother
Are you there?
Do you hear me?
No, because the voices prevail
Hello my brother
Can you breathe?
The air inside your lungs
Strangles you indeed
Hello my brother
No, they are not after you
But one thousand times
It's said
Imaginary people
Deep inside your head
Hello my brother
It's me
I was there when you were small
I remember you at 15
Hello my brother,
The voices
The sounds
The screams, the fear
We couldn't buy your friends
They wouldn't stay near!
They didn't understand
The gifts that you have
Hello my brother
When daddy died
We tried to manage the best we could
To that
We would divide
Goodnight my brother
May the voices disappear
You are my only brother

I wish you were not who you are
In the sense of all of your scars
How I knew when you were
A baby
Stolen and replaced
With someone else

BROKEN PHONE

So glad you answered
He said to me
My phone is broken
And I am scared
No, hon, we are speaking, it's ok
I will always be there
Will you call me tomorrow?
Yes, I will
The phone kept ringing
Don't be scared
I'll keep trying

BELIEVE WHAT I TELL YOU

The dogs are chasing after me
They ripped my pants
Began to pee
They barked a lot
Pushed me in the street
I looked down and said
To myself
These are not my feet
They're yours
Don't tell me different
The voices, the voices
It's real
I see it

ONCE 32

Teeth that is
One by one
Chipping away
Being pulled
They've had their day
Toothbrush
In place
Never used
No encouragement
Lots of discouragement
No family
To get out of
The haze
To encourage
To care for your health
So, you hide your smile
For the empty hole
Is minus the white
Full of cavities
And pain
The resistance of
Care
Not in your rein

THE BOSS AND I

I think you are dyslexic
"Well I think you lack common sense!"

YOU TOUCH PEOPLE'S HEARTS

You asked me why I said
You touch people's hearts
Simply put,
Your heart is pure!

SATURDAY MORNING

My brother and I
Playing downstairs
Making noise
It didn't blare
My mother came
But not to play
Dressed us up
Locked us outside
We kicked and kicked
To be let in
Seems like it went on for hours
Until finally
She had her rest
And we were able to go back to the warmth
Of a home?

LABELS

Labels
Titles and more
Determine
Where we've been
And where we might explore
Am I smart?
Am I not?
You can't, you won't
Don't fight it
We have been labeled!

DON'T SPY ON ME

I finally reached you by phone today
You explained
You were upset that
I was calling people to spy on you
I was worried
I will try to not do that again
But I too panic
I'm unable to keep my feelings in check
You are my family
Your deck of cards
Has become mine
Forever, we will align

WHO IS THAT GUY WALKING DOWN THE STREET?

I came to visit
You weren't home
Got in the car
To search for you
Back and forth
The street you travel
Finally found you
Hoodie on, head down
My heart ached
Why you?
Why you?
You could have been spared
When you saw me, you glared
And then your eyes smiled
You got into the car
Drove back to your
Apartment
It wasn't too far
I wanted to hold
Tightly for a long while
You have your own style
Of love and release
I'll cherish the moments
Forever
And pray for your peace

SHADOWS IN MY MIND

Shadows creeping everywhere
Is it true?
Are they there?
Don't you see them?
I want to share
The sights I see
Hard to bare
I can't explain
How my mind works
Everything I see
Is real to me
I wish I didn't
Why can't they let me be?

CLOSET ABOVE THE BATHTUB

The closet was a scary place
My brother would
Hide and not show his face
His illness
Proved different ways to think
And share
Yet underneath
Fear was there
His smile
Would change
In a single second
That fear of unknown
That always mentioned

THE VIRUS

I know you feel abandoned
It's not my choice at all
The COVID
Which you fear
Prevents our touch
And to be near
I give my word
Soon
I'll clean the floor
Hug your head
Remind you that all your family
Is not dead

I WAS LOVED

Mom and Dad loved me
They did everything they could
Didn't they?
I wasn't easy to live with
I miss them
They too were different!

PIZZA

Every Day I go for pizza
Two slices and a drink
I pay $5.00
That's pretty good, you think?
I have to walk a mile
To get to the store
And sometimes
It's hard on me
My health is failing
Some days I don't go outside
I eat some cereal
That's what I have
Will you send me Halvah?
Thank you

DON'T YOU SEE THEM?

I want to share
The sights I live
Hard to bare
I can't explain
How my mind works
Everything I see
Is real to me
I wish I didn't
Why can't they let me be?

DEER IN THE WOODS

I love the deer
Next to my apartment
In the Woods
Innocent
They want love
Just like me
Do you see the babies, following their mom?
I like to watch them
They bring me peace
Better than people
They don't bite
Just want to be fed
And stay in their home
The Woods
They can freely roam
Better than humans

My brother Wrote This

When a man has
Fear in him he has
nougting But when a man
has courage he has
quieted the storm.

I DIDN'T MEAN IT

I'm sorry
I didn't mean it
I'm sick
I can't help it
I love you
I wish you were still here
It's ok, I understand you
I will never abandon you
I will be back
Don't apologize
I get it
My love will never stop
Please know as long as I am breathing
I will return

"When a man is stubborn he falls to his knees
A man with common sense will find his own way"

My brother

THUNDER IN MY VOICE

Did you know Thunder's not in the sky?
It's in the bones
Of when I cry
Screams of horror
Uncertainty
Fear
Terrified they might take me away
From those that are near
The thunder is fierce
It speaks to the voices
A battle immense
It doesn't make sense
And provides no choices

THE POLICE

The police are after me
The dogs are here
No they're not!
He knows what he saw
The blood in his veins
No friends
No enemies
Just him

I CAN HARDLY WALK

It's hard to walk
I cannot bend
To the store
I travel
It's a dead-end

MOON RIVER

The darkness of life
Surrounds a man I know
He can't make a sound
A secret he hides
So deep inside
Others know
But don't understand
The fear subsides
He cries alone
A mere moan
A Childhood that never existed
The voices have always persisted
The teen years vanished with the blink of an eye
So many tears
He lost all of his years
The cruelness of peers
Still he has fears
He can't express
The very being of existence
We knows he feels
And tries to hide
The demons inside
This man I know
My brother
The song "Moon River"
Brought tears to his eyes
The depth of his soul
Never rose to be noticed
He's still a man
A human being
Warm and deserving
To be healed
From his bleeding
(Paranoid Schizophrenia is like a cancer that goes on for a
lifetime)

BUY ME

She would pay!
My mothers' gift to you
Would be my brother
For a day

Some things can't be bought
Some people, no one wants
Tragic as it seems
That's a life
With absolutely no good dreams

TEMPLATE

No template
No pattern
No structure
No matter
No Vision
No grandeur
No living
No answer
Voices
Instructing
A lack of control
Continue enhancing
The darkness within
His very soul

Chapter 2: Myself

I'm NOT Schizophrenic but I have a bit of crazy

"He always wanted to be someone's whole world forever! He is!"

Francine Fuentes

HOODIE

Cold or Warm
Your face is covered
Within your hoodie
You mask your face
Your sparkling eyes
They can't erase
Do people
Know you're not alone?
You belong to family
And spent nights in a home?
That you are loved
But do they care?
Can they see beyond
Your disheveled hair?
Common sense they lack the most
They mock, ignore
And believe they're immune
It's random, how the mind goes
Could be at birth
Or in their teens
Elderly and in between
BE KIND – ISOLATION KILLS

"Compassion, empathy and a good heart are the best ways to prove one is educated"

Francine Fuentes

THE CRAZY LAUGHTER

With a burst of noise
Like a cannonball
With a boom
The crazy laugh
I ask
Myself
What tickles your heart
We don't know
It fills the room
The crazy laugh
Contagious at times
It's great to hear
The sound
From your belly
As it's rare
To see joy
Come from your throat
And then turn to jelly

WHO IS CRAZY?

"I was told by a school counselor that I could never do more than work at McDonald's REALLY?.... I can't believe you are an educator!" My brother receives more of the same!
Francine Fuentes

THE BUTTER DISH

We would save all our pennies
To make you both happy
My brother and I would
Walk to the store
And buy a butter dish
For 25 cents
No more
We would beam with pride
And bring it inside
To buy the love
A quarter could bribe

BREATHE

Inhalers are all over the place
On the small table
On the couch by your side
Next to your feet
They are empty
Your lungs have used them up
You say you need more
You can't do without!
You won't be able to breathe
With no air in the spout
You say this will kill you
Without a doubt
My baby brother
Breathe!

LATCH ON

I searched for love
Throughout my childhood life
And made choices
That caused so much strife
Begging for love
Latching on
To save me
From what I was born
A good girl I was
And pleased above and beyond
Didn't realize what was ahead or behind
Sorry
Thank you
I will
Until I am dead
Is confidence eaten away in your brain
From living unhappy?

MY BROTHER SITTING ON THE SIDEWALK

Your head hung low
You are my blood
Watching you alone
Breaks my heart
Breaks the rules of
How a humans life should not be
Why the good people?
Why you?
I want us to have a healthy life together
I want to hold your head up
I want you to feel joy
My brother, I am your sister
When you hurt, I suffer
I want to make you better.

SILENCE

Deep in conversation
On the phone
Seconds of laughter
You aren't alone
Things going smoothly
Then silence sets in
Are you there?
Everything's quiet
I ask again
Then we hang up.

HOUSE OF HORROR

My mom
Loving
As much as she could
Her life a horror
I understood
She hid from herself
Flashing in and out of ours
My brother not there
Invisible
It seemed
She often left
I didn't know why
But remember
The screaming
The threats
He could not help
But possessed
The power of control
Yet he didn't know it
My brother
Schizophrenic
It became our normal

THE TELEPHONE SHOOK

The night before my baby was born
The phone call came
With a powerful storm
Threats towards my baby
The jealousy set in
I hung up the phone
With blanket over my head
And began to feel that horrible dread

I'M SICK

Mom, my stomach hurts
I can't go to school
The pain is bad
I'm sick all the time
Let me stay home and
Just plain sleep
To hide from the fear
So very deep
I'm too young
To carry the burdens
I can't think at school
And can't even learn
The kids make fun of me
Each and every day
I smell
My clothes are torn
Please let me stay home
And hide from the world
I'm just a child
I want to be your little girl

THE WINDOW

Through the window
He slithered inside
To hide from my brother
Who would tell
Not deny
My mother
Would shelter
As anyone would
I had no friends
Just imaginary
To keep me company
As I could only do wrong
My brother
My little one
He was very strong

LESSONS IN LEARNING

Don't judge
Don't say we can't
Don't say – do it my way!
Don't downplay
Don't erase ideas
Don't erase history
What I could not do at 5 – no longer matters
What I could not do at 10 – no longer matters
What I could not do at 15 – no longer matters
What I could not do at 21 – no longer matters
What I could not do at 60 – no longer matters
What I could not do
NO LONGER MATTERS!
My brother and I matter!

THE EMPTY HOUSE

Hiding in closets
Behind closed doors
Waiting for eruption
Of my brothers roar
He had no control
We were all full of sadness
To watch a young boy
Fight off his madness
Our mother was lost
Amidst all the fury
So sometimes
She left for days at a time
To find the relief
She tried hard to find
Acceptance was null
Her son…so very ill
His brain couldn't make
The pieces stay still
Picked up the remnants
And as long as I could
I tried to improve
The household of heartache
To this day
We are empty
For our brother now grown
The childhood lost
There are no more words
But at what cost
Schizophrenia tore
Down the walls of
Our brother

HOMELESS IN PHILLY

Homeless in a Beautiful Setting
Philadelphia, PA
A peaceful setting by the river
Couples mulling around
One woman sleeping on a bench
Visitors walking by
As if she was not there
I think of my brother
How he feels
Singled out
Might be a good thing
Instead
Of
Pretending someone is not there!

COVERED FURNITURE

Torn sheets
Strewn across
The sofa
Torn sheets
Across each and every chair
I tried to make it nice
But no one was there
Torn sheets
Stuffed in the side of seats
So friends would think our home was pretty
To cover all the pain
Torn sheets
Were in my control
That's where I was vain
And tried to play the role
In charge, I was not
But pretending kept me going
Like a very tight knot
Yet inside my stomach
I often felt like rotted wood
That needs to be polished
To shine
Be neat
And uncovered

THRILLER

I remember
Dancing with my brother
To Thriller
The only girl that was there
I remember
Travels to Philly
His face would light up
For just a moment
His expression
Would often change
I knew at that moment
He could become deranged
The moods, the demons
Inside my brother
There was no script
It would just occur
The darkness of his eyes
Schizophrenia
Always as it were
A disease we learned to despise

FENDING

Walking home
From school
My brother in hand
Children didn't understand
They would kick he and I
As we walked to our home
I would try to protect
So he wouldn't feel alone
So home we traveled
Yet when we arrived
We were alone
To fend for ourselves
No one was there
He would often shove me
Push me
He ruled the house
I don't blame you my brother
Destiny

THE BOY

He noticed me on the stairs of my high school
I was happy
He saw me
I was someone
I had no idea of the fear he soon instilled in me
Throwing me down the stairs
Of his mothers' home
Was it so terrible?
I kept going back
Home was not where I wanted to be
So again and again
He would take me back
I wanted to escape
I wanted to be saved!

MEAT GRINDER

As a current day vegetarian
I can't believe this happened!
My father grinding beef
On the dining room table
My brother and I
Hands cupped below
To shove
Uncooked meat into our mouths
I think this was a happier moment??

"Sometimes people with a big heart sketched on their arm can be the most heartless."

Francine Fuentes

FOG

Much more than
Blur
Fuzz
Mist in the air
It's the capacity
To be aware
It's a heart
That wants to heal
Fighting what is real
Break through the fog
The gray that blocks
The haze in my mind
That can't declare
It's ok
When it's not
The pain is there
The fog, the chill
Emptiness

LOST

Does God look down
And see lost souls?
Together led
Some are dead
Does God look down at
Fleeting Souls
Natures must
Does God look down
And laugh at us
Whisper softly
You are but dust

HOUSE OF SAD

My mom
Loving
As much as she could
Her life a horror
I understood
She hid from herself
By flashing in and out of others
My brother not there
Invisible
It seemed
She often left
I didn't know why
But remember
The screaming
The threats
He could not help
But possessed
The power of control
Yet he didn't know it
My brother
Schizophrenic
The new normal

DON'T BE LONELY

Please don't abandon me
 You're my brother
I don't want you to hurt
You deserve all that's good
You've been dealt a bad hand
I pray to God that
Soon you will land
On your feet where
You were planted
My brother, my heart
Don't hurt
Don't be lonely
I will be back
Until then
Freeze the panic attack

DEATH

When someone dies
We lose a piece of ourselves
Yet, the burden is buried
Is that ok to say?

TAKE IT

You like my dress
Well, here it is
You like my shoes
They're yours, not his
You like my ring
Take it now
Do you like me?
Or what I give
Clothes, my stuff
Or what I hid
Starving
For a friend like you
I'm running out of
Things to do
Little left for me, myself
Take it all
It's on the shelf
When you return
With closed hands
Then I'll know
Our
Friendship
Will
Grow

ON THE ROAD TO ATLANTIC CITY

I remember you telling stories of
Driving your car to Atlantic City,
The Poconos
Wildwood, NJ
You felt free
You described the freedom
Of being on the road
Just you and Buddy
You have a wonderful sense of direction
I wish I were like you
I get lost between home
And my workplace
Wish I were smart like you
You appreciate the sand
The water
The sky
The snow
In your eyes
When your mind is clear
You see beauty in seashells and stars
The gauge on your card reads O
You kept going
You and your Buddy
The sky you see is brighter than any of us could imagine
You have expressed this so many times
I wish I could drive with you to Atlantic City
And share the beauty you feel in your heart
I love you sweetie

THE ROOF OVER YOUR HEAD

I'm glad there is a roof
That keeps you safe at night
The door has a lock
It's your small haven
The walls are bare
No decorations
I want to make it your home

IF TREES COULD SPEAK

If trees could speak
They'd say to you
Your heart
Shapes branches, leaves and vines
You see the earth
With depth, few know
Your love of nature
When wind glazes over grass
Respect of
Rabbits, deer and furry things
Your mind
Brings truth
For all small things
You're on this earth
To plant YOUR seeds
Your heart will live
Through the trees
That will be here for a hundred years
They'll speak of you
Your soft heart
Remembering the man
With greatest respect
For their forest
They will not forget
Schizophrenia brings greater descriptions of beauty

"Grab scissors and cut out the bad, then create the most spectacular pattern of your life."

Francine Fuentes

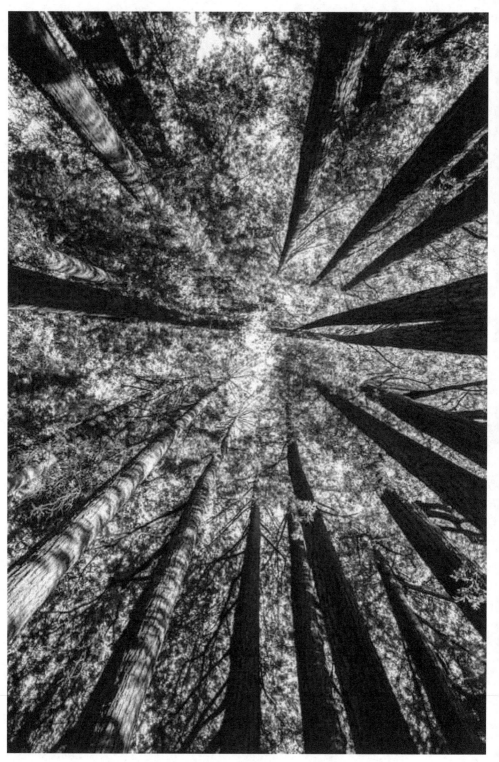

HAPPY BIRTHDAY TO YOU

Alone you are
Waiting for what?
A card in the mail?
A knock at your door?
A phone call
Will you answer just once more?
Will your neighbors be kind?
When family's not there
Will the voices
Tell you that we truly care?
Will you rest tonight?
One year older
Feel warm
And no older
Will you dream
Of the time
Before you were born
And pray
Your future
Will be so much more?

I AM WHAT I SAW

I became what I learned
What I saw
What I heard
What I observed
The pit
Of my being
Often disturbed
Out of control
Many of my days
The childhood lost
Often makes
Time a haze
When I want to bury
The sadness and worry
I wonder who will be there
To take care of me
As I with my brother
My mother
My family of three
My sibling would move on
As she was of age
That too is a haze
My brother
My turn
Yesterday
And so the fears carry on with my own
That was born to me
Scared to let go
And so I want to be
The mother who can accept
What will be will be
No difference, my brother
My mother
The family of three

"Is it easier to be left than leave."

Francine Fuentes

A STRING OF CLEANER

I bought you a new mop
So that I could clean your floors
Inspection is coming up
And I want to be sure
Hey, my mop is gone
Someone has taken it from me
My brother, no one would take your mop
But I checked and checked
And surely it was gone
Is it his mind telling him stories
Or is true
The voices do implore
That there might or might not even be a floor

EDUCATION

What isn't taught in school
Is to be kind and nurture the mind
For those that don't have a voice
To provide a voice for those that need one
To see the future
And provide direction
For those that don't follow the same road
To instill hope
To not demean
To understand
To see beauty in the
Third side of the mind
Has this even been discovered?
It's your job
To not judge
It's your job
To nudge!
It saddens me
You don't have a clue
In your safe little world
Until it affects you!

I'M A GOOD CLEANER MOMMY

I cleaned the kitchen
When 5 years old
My mother came home
And to her admission
Said something mean
I cried
On my hands and knees
The love I wanted
I begged to please
Not clean enough
I love you mom
Love me back!

I WONDER

Is mental illness
From down under?
If one has it
Then do we all?
Is it random
In the genes?
Or from a fall?
We all hear voices
From within
But are they demons?
Or just a whim
Are we all a bit off?
Are we all sane?
I think a mixture
Is more correct
Learning to live
With what comes
And living
With no name

SICK OF

My stomach hurts
Can't go to school
My throat is scratchy
I'm just too ill
To school I'd go
And my neighbor
Always there
To bring me home
And serve me tea and toast
I felt loved
My neighbor,
Thank you for being there.
I'll never forget your name
You were the strength
And allowed me to be a child
For a moment in time
But then seemed like a great while
The row home in Philly
Two doors away
I could go there at any time to
Be a child for a day

MYSELF THE MOTHER

I try to undo the worst of me
Protect my son
Til he can't breathe
I meant the best
Inside of me
I love him so
I realize I must let go
So he can be the person
He's meant to be
And not follow
The life of
ME
He's full of life
Perfect as he is
He will never be the parent
To his parent!

"Why are you mean to those that can't fight back? Do you get pleasure from this act?"

Francine Fuentes

DROP OUT

He didn't drop out of school
Because he wasn't good enough
He dropped out
Because he was too smart
Felt more than most
He was different
Kids can be heartless
Learned from adults
He is my brother
He is someone's son!

" If more people would drop in, less would drop out."

Francine Fuentes

NOT SO EASY

Thin? Eat more!
Overweight? Stop eating?
Shy? Speak Louder!
Slow at Learning? Learn Faster!
Ill? Be well!
Alone? Find someone!
Homeless? Buy a home!
Depressed? Snap out of it!
Mentally ill? Don't be!
Not so easy!

BE KIND! BE BETTER! BE HUMAN!

"Often, those that have a home are homeless."

Francine Fuentes

DEAR BROTHER

If I could rip through your brain
Kill the disease
Reverse all your pain
I want to ease
Anguish you feel
Day in and out
Your beautiful heart
Stifled with fear
What can I do?
I want to be near
You're under attack
A foreign body
We don't know
What is it?
I am so sorry
I love you
I love you
I hate all your pain
Normal, what is that?
To be sane? Like others???

DEMONS RULE HIS WORLD

They demand
He listens
Control every thought
They travel through microwaves,
Toilet and door
Sometimes they seek him out
When sleeping on the floor
They speak
In other languages
A variety of sounds
They paralyze with fearsome voice
And crumble to the ground
They take him where he shouldn't go
He can't fight
They are stronger than he
Deliberate and monstrous
They see his weakness
Break his brain
It's not him, it's them
That's insane!
Finally, they flee!

PHILLY BASEMENT

Junk, cartons of photos,
I can't relate
Old piano
Took lessons
Afraid
Of the creepy darkness
Hated practice
My brother would push me in
And lock the door
Looking down was frightening
The light turned off from the other side
Terrified of
The scary people
That could be below
The floor
And the other side of the door

WAKE UP AND SMELL THE MESS!

Sugarcoat all I want
Perfect parents, perfect life
Overrated!
Understated!
I survived!

FIFTY-FIVE JOBS

At the very least
Smart as he was
Never given a chance
To prove he could
They judged by a glance
Not fitting the mold
That gets old
People forget
It could be them
A father
A mother
A sister
A brother
It hits when
Not looking
A second it takes
For life to be
Different
Like pushing a rake
Inside the brain
The pain is hidden
The jobs
For him
Always forbidden

SOMEONE'S SON

My brother
Is someone's son
He had a mother and father
 Pretty messed up!
People avoid
Eye contact
To make him go away

His illness did not destroy
His heart
He is someone's son
He came from somewhere
God brought him here
He belongs
He doesn't need flowers
When he's gone
But NOW,
He needs Smiles, a sandwich
A cheerful hello
Goes a long way
While he's breathing
My brother
He's a human being
He will always be someone's son

THE SQUEEZE

The squeeze
Searching for love
Wanting to please
Too much,
Too fast,
Too hard,
Won't last
Parent, sibling, sometimes a boss
Similarities
But know
In that
We want
Approval
Why fight so hard
When in a moment
Work harder, faster
Dim, and then darker
Finally
Light is gone
Even longer
Stifled we are
The mind is not free
Let it be
We aren't who they think
Do they care?

AGE OF THREE

You beat me up
Your strength
Hurt me
A baby
Made me black and blue
Kicking my legs
They said
It's OK
That's what boys do!

KISSES

I slowly approach
While you're sitting down
Your head hangs low
Your hoodie
Envelops your face
No eye contact
You smile meekly
When I kiss your cheek
Body tenses
You are so sweet
You need love
So do I !
Please let me fix this!
I owe it to you

"Mommy, we hated when you left us. We felt abandoned! We haven't recovered."

Francine Fuentes

"Saying goodbye means I no longer have that sick knot in my stomach."

Francine Fuentes

WHY THE HELL WERE WE LEFT ALONE?

Mommy,
Where were you?
Why were we left alone?
What the hell were you thinking?

A COMMON PHONE CALL

You Whore!
You Bitch!
I hope you f..ing die
Don't call me again
You lie
You never do anything for me!
That's how it will be
And then the comments continue
He hangs up or I do…
I know this isn't him
It's the illness
Within
The deep dark voices
Frustrations
Coping and lack of
Battling himself
The World
His being
The tears
Keep streaming

"Guilt Comes Easy To Me, I've earned a Certificate of Guilt!"

Francine Fuentes

THE KITCHEN IS CLEAN

Five years old I cleaned the kitchen
Mommy came home
And to her admission
Said something derogatory
I then cried and cried
On my hands and knees
The love I wanted
I often begged to please

ASPIRIN

He broke up with me
I couldn't cope
To the aspirin bottle
I traveled
With very little hope
I wanted to sleep
Aspirin was weak
But on the hospital bed
My dad showed up with tears
What have you done?
I explained my fears
I'm alone
The boy left me
I wasn't enough
I'd rather die
Than be alone
Aspirin was a waste
Yes, I tried in haste

BAR MITZVAH

I'm sad, I missed
Your special day
I wasn't there
It's late
But
I want you to know
I am sorry
But very proud
You earned the pomp and circumstance
Of achieving this milestone
Yet in your heart
Always alone
I wish it could be a do-over

BECAUSE OF YOU

I'm called a mom
Because of you
I took the leap
Because of you
I learned how
Because of you
 I Followed through
Because of you
We have our own family
Thank you

BED OF SPRINGS

You slept on a bed of springs
No one knew
Except for you
No blanket to cover
The sofa was hard
And not long enough
You slept huddled
In your secret place
With voices
That tell you things
You try to erase
Sleeping alone
No dog by your side
Your bones are brittle
It's hard to stand up
Yet you can carry on
For many of the same ahead
Full of voices, so much dread

WHY ARE YOU LOOKING AT ME FUNNY?

Why are you looking at me the way that you do?
I see it, I know and you do too!
Your face looks weird
I don't like what you're doing
Get out of my house!
I don't want you here
Don't come back!
Leave now!
Do you hear?
The Paranoia sets in.

TORTURED BROTHER

Meds
Keep you going
But also take you away
The joy you might feel
Is different each day
The hospital you were taken to
Was cold, damp and sad
I wanted to protect you
From the insanity that surrounded
Everyone who stayed there
Yet, once you escaped
To be brought back again
With those
They treated opposite
Of the human race
But you are different
You are my brother
I am sorry

"We can be born into, grow out of and become extraordinarily creative."

Francine Fuentes

" Brain activity is altered. Love us for who we are, that's all we can be."

Francine Fuentes

BROKEN TEETH

My two front teeth
Broke on ice
They stayed
That way for years
My parents didn't fix them then
I was sad with tears
To school I'd travel
Hand over mouth
When I spoke, I mumbled
So they would not see
The ugly girl
That shout at me
I turned 18
They were fixed
My hand dropped down
My smile appeared
Different than how I was raised
A completed smile
I embraced.
The homely girl

MILESTONES LOST

No engagement
No marriage
No children carry your name
No parties
No graduation
Invisible birthday's
No celebration
No anticipation
Each day is the same
Why does God
Randomly choose
Who will win, and who will lose?
You are more deserving
Than anyone I know
I love you!

PANIC ATTACK

One hour, 5 or 24
The worst feeling to ever endure
He can't breathe
Muscles contract
His back aches
His legs are weak
Tunnel vision
Attack
Ready, set, go
The always come back
Whenever they choose
Not his choice
For he will always lose

"You can't schedule an appointment with Mental illness."

Francine Fuentes

SELF DESTRUCTION

If he could push a button
To end it all
It would be with music
His favorite song
He remembers so many
So damn smart
Why can't we fix it?
Destroy the bad records
Inside his brain
And replace with
A mixture
Of his favorites
A heartwarming twist
To rid
The demons
And drown them with sound
That's happy
And soothing
Rescue him NOW!

"Compassion, empathy and a good heart are the best ways to prove one is educated."

Francine Fuentes

CALL THE DOCTOR

Can you trust them?
Are they true?
Will they be quiet
When you speak
Keep their word
When you weep
Give you meds
Or send you on?
Keep your confidence
Or sell your soul
I pray they are human
And have children of their own
So they treat with respect
After we're gone

CRAVING KIWI

As my mother lay on her bed
Her final days
She asked for Kiwi
Then a beer
Finally, came my brother's name
I wanted to ignore
I promised
I would care for him
As I did when I was young
Inside frightened
If that came true
How my life would be un-done
My mother passed
My brother alone
I'm sorry mommy
I needed my OWN!

CRAZY

I think we all are
In some way
Is it genetic?
Is it just the day?
Is it what I learned?
Maybe a gift from God
Think about great artists and authors
Who were labeled more often than not!
Did they write from the heart?
Did they paint on the easel?
Or hear and see images
Without a special place
The voices may tell us
It's time to NOT erase
Our thoughts
And practices
Are who we are
Sometimes it's good
To carry a creative scar!

DANCER

Look Mom,
I can dance
That can be my job
As I would prance
I don't need math
Or scientific measures
Just graceful limbs
That YOU will treasure
I began to teach
And loved that job
For the moment,
I was great
Still
I wasn't enough

ABANDONMENT

Please don't abandon me
I promise, I won't
You are my brother
I don't want you to hurt
You deserve all that's good
You've been dealt a bad hand
I pray to God that
Soon you will land
On your feet
You were planted here
My brother, my heart
Don't hurt
Don't be lonely
I will be back
Until then
Freeze the panic attack

DON'T CHECK ON ME

You answered the phone, this time
You answered
You explained
You were upset that
I was calling people to check on you
I was worried
I will try to not do that again
But I too panic
I'm unable to keep my feelings in check
You are my family
Your deck of cards
Has become mine
Forever, we will align

EAT THE MEAT

Beef was cooked, or whatever it was
Eat it now
I tried to swallow
But would gag
From the smell of blood
And the texture
From the hollow
You will eat it
Later today!
Oh, my stomach was sick
If I could feed
Sleepy, our dog on the sly
It was a good day
Our dog would save our brother and I

EXORCISM

Remember the movie
When evil was removed
By a ritual
Induced by
Someone with power
That rid all of the pain
Consistent for hours
My mom and I
Spoke of the last try
To remove the devil
If one existed
The sadness
Inside
The house
That wept
When my brother cried
And screamed with pain
We wanted to hide
Inside the drain
He needed us
So here we are
Nothing has changed
The process was not completed
So, we did retreat

HOME MADE CIGARETTES

While visiting you in your apartment
I cleaned that day
And in the drawer were contraptions
I had not seen before
To make home-made cigarettes
To calm you down
I threw them out
So You'd stay well
That didn't work
So, what the hell!
Everyone has a vice
You deserve
So much more
Cigarettes
Calm you
I won't as before

EYES

Eyes don't deceive
They evolve into
Happy
They turn into sad
They close
When you are thinking
They smile
When you're glad
They tear
When you are frightened
Alone inside your heart
Heavy when you're tired
The lines became so deep
Your life
Has so much meaning
Your eyes somewhat bleak
The sparkle
Left you
Like when I'm off my meds
They are after me

FETAL POSITION

Throughout my life
The fetal position
 Saved me
Tightly curled into a ball
No one could reach me
Let me sleep!
Please close the door
A trance I chose
To not feel pain
The small curled body
The Thoughts
Feelings
Emptiness
I felt
With family
Boys
Not fitting in
I needed love
I had thin skin

FIRST BATH

Encouragement
To do simple tasks
Such as bathe himself
Not so easy!
Not sure how
His trust for our cousin
Brought soap to his body
With water
And foam
A step most
Don't understand
Unless they are alone
Mental illness
Brings phobias of all kinds
Not an easy feat
Parts unspoken
The body feels better
Relief of some sort
Thank you my cousin
For being more
Than a sport
This trend has been broken
Cleaner he was
Soap and water
Will last a long time

FLUTTERS

That feeling of doom in my core
The ill feelings reoccur
Insecurities
My parents often not there
My brother and I
Too much to bare
Responsibilities
Protective of him
Yet I wanted my childhood freedom
To be whom I might be
And not hiding in the shadows
Of what I was born into
My brother
I loved him and still do
However, he became my son
And I was too young
To be the one

FRIENDS REMEMBER

After searching many years
Found a friend from way back when
We spoke, we laughed
And remembered then
We were kids
And spoke of our
Moms and dads
And houses we compared
I liked hers
She liked mine
I asked her why
Then she mentioned
My brother
And his life
She remembers
There was something
Different
An enormous amount of strife
Quiet with no life

FROZEN IN TIME

Body Stops!
As do brains
When lack of something
Will not retain
Thoughts
Of that human cell
To make them
Stay in a living hell
Mental illness
The secrets
Stay behind the walls
Of hell
Unless a guest
Pops in unexpectedly
And unmasks
The truth of our family

HE SAID

I wish mom and dad
Were still here
I'm afraid
To be without them
Better when they were near
What if I get sick?
Who'll take care of me?
Mom would always hug me
Dad would buy me cars
I miss them so much
I get scared
Do you hear me?
Are you there?

HIS WORDS

"When a man has fear in him he has nothing,
but when a man has courage he has quieted the storm."

I JUST REMEMBERED

Memories of my mom, brother and I watching *The Flintstones* on Friday nights. I would walk to an ice cream store in Philadelphia, purchase three cones of ice cream and old fashioned pretzels to bring home for our big night. By the time I would reach our small row home, the ice cream would be dripping down my arms....
Happy moment

I'M NOT ENOUGH

I love you
I don't
Be this way
Or I won't
You are stupid!
You won't amount to anything!
So just don't bother
But I will
I'm lonely
You know
I just want a small house
With a picket fence to call my own
It was never enough
I still love you my mother and father
You died way too young
To see what I've become
I hope you can see me from up above
And know that I'm a woman
That has grown over the top!
And still overcoming
The past of no childhood
I love you
And always will
Please give me a sign
I look at your photos still

INHALER

Your inhalers are all over the place
On the small table
On the couch by your side
Next to your feet
They are empty
Your lungs have used them up
You say you need more
You can't do without!
You won't be able to breathe
With no air in the spout

LET'S CLEAN THE HOUSE AND WE WILL BE PERFECT

I'll fill the bucket
You pick up the rest
I'll scrub each step
On the staircase
Towards her bed
And make it shine
Please just a moment
Do not cry or whine
Let's make toast
And bring hot tea
A loving note
From you and me
To mommy's bed
She will feel like a princess
And love us more
I was a little girl
And you a little boy
We did good together
Creating love
Cleaning the floor
And then when asked
We'd close the door

LITTLE SELF

She tried to find
A piece of you
Tucked away
In smiles
And pleasing
And lost herself
While searching
So hard
Little self
You were five years old
Not a mother, father
Barely able to hold on

6TH GRADE

School counselor
And parents
"Your daughter is lovely"
BUT, the best she will be able to do is
Work at McDonald's!
I believed her!!!!!!
Who is mentally ill?
 She could have stopped me!
What if I believed her forever?
What if my brother had a chance?

"Mental illness is so screwed up! But so are we!"

Francine Fuentes

MISSING MY MOTHER

Mostly, I saw you once a year
You came to California
You were a breath of fresh air
What I loved most was
Sitting on my sofa
Holding your hand
Talking for hours
About your dreams
For me to move on to
A new life
And how difficult yours was
I wanted you to have more happy moments
And feel the ocean breeze
California
I wanted to please
I know you loved me with all your heart
But often fell off the chart
We are a product of our past
My memories of you
Have all come back
You loved me mommy
And I still love you

MOODY

Happy
Unsure
Too sure
Disheveled
How I turned out from my dysfunctional family
They did the best they could
And, so did I
So here I am at 63
Still asking why
My brain is so tangled, all not connected
Yet creativity
Saves me
To that I was selected

MY BROTHERS' BIRTHDAY

He received 3 birthday cards from neighbors
One had candy
Another had treats
They are nice people, he said
They check on me
Some weeks
It makes me sad
That you are basically alone
With each passing birthday
Your heart is empty
But beautiful

SEE ME

Woke up in the morning
A knot so tight
I couldn't breathe
Chose to stay in bed
And not be the lead
I wanted to be a child
But my role was chosen for me
To care for my parents
And younger brother
Or else they would ignore me
Rather than explore me

OREO COOKIES

I'd hide in room
Lock my door
Marriage of hell
The cookies
Became
My very best friend
Under the covers
I'd eat a whole box
It filled the emptiness
Of marriage
Unhinged
As my mind slowly went to waste
The sugar inside
Filled the void
Of loneliness
In California
I died

"Our brother will always be our little brother."

Francine Fuentes

PAPER DOLLS

The middle room
I'd scatter paper
Scissors in hand
I'd draw smiling faces
With wide eyes
A man
A Woman
Children
A room with books
The kitchen was warm
With lots of hooks
I'd cut the people figures
In similar ways
They'd sit all day
Smiling at each other
And then a hug
My family of figures
My dreams
Would they finally come?

PLASTIC CONTAINER FULL OF PENNIES

Hundreds of pennies in a box
Under the table on the floor
Along with small rocks
One of your rituals
I see one peeking from underneath the rug
Still another and more
I help to drop them in the box
So the vacuum won't eat them
Along with the dust, crumbs of food
And other debris
Paper wrappers
Juice boxes
And more
Not enough time to remove
And explore
But you will know
What has been touched
It's your safety net
Perhaps for a rainy day
I know that much
There is more rain than sun for you

PNEUMONIA

The social worker
Called to say
Your brothers ill
This time
In a different way
His breathings labored
Oxygen attached
He has no strength
He wants you to come back
Alone he was
So sad for him
Our reality
I despised
He was alone
I arrived at his apartment
My cousin joined me
And that made it
Better
He recovered for now
Who knows what's next
This illness is a continuous test!

POSSESSED

When my mom passed away
Furniture and trinkets followed me to my Denver home
Unpacked and felt somewhat alone
A photo in an ornate frame
Was left downstairs
On a table
The middle of the night
We felt unsettled
My husband and I awakened
With fright
The photo instructed us
To remove it from the house
We ran downstairs
And took it to out
Into the trash, it would reside
Not sure
What happened
But it was real
Unsettling to say the least
Mommy, you loved me
The message was not meek
Afterwards, we were able to sleep

PSYCHOLOGISTS NEVER GO OUT OF BUSINESS

Someone to talk to
Vent to
Listen to
They can be productive
Some are effective
Like all professions
Some should not be
But when you find
A good one
That cares
Stay a while!
Talk about your past
Your future
Write a book!

THE REWARD

Growing up hearing "you can't"
Stay home
Handle this and handle that
On May 16th
I celebrated what is to me
A major feat
I proudly walked across the stage
At Tropicana Field
And met a goal
So this is my new age
No parents on hand
Not even my brother
Wish they could hold my hand
And say
Mazel Tov

SKILLET ON THE FLOOR

Burned food on the skillet
On the floor it remains
Remnants of your meal that day
Or a week with thick film
It seems to be the same
Can you put it on the table?
No, it's ok where it is
I want you safe
I try to follow the rules
To protect you
I'm not there every day
So if the skillet
Stays in place
The floor
Your kitchen counter
It really is your space

SKYDIVING

In my thirties
I explored the sky
Quite a feat
For heights is not
A favorite of I
I called my mom
To brag a bit
She got angry
Hung up the phone
Called me stupid
I tried to call back
I felt alone
Several days went by
When she answered my call
She was worried
That I might fall
I was trying to prove
To myself and others
I was brave
And wanted encouragement
From my parent
To save
This incredible memory
I had created
I didn't mean to frighten
I was simply elated

SOLVE THE PROBLEM

Mrs. Teacher, I can't
Then you will stand at the Blackboard
Until you do
A soft whisper
"I don't understand"
What don't you understand, she asked?
Anything
Stand here until you do
I never understood
Why the punishment
Was so great
And why
That teacher
Sought to
Berate
I hate to imagine how my brother was treated in school!

"I always wanted to be someone's whole world forever!"

Francine Fuentes

"Sometimes people with a big heart can be the most heartless"

Francine Fuentes

STILLNESS

When I was still
I'd hide under the covers
No one could see me
Invisible as night
The darkness
Would take away the fright....
Of where I belonged
And where I did not
My home was empty
Like shattered glass
It didn't matter
Get through the day
No matter which way
Opposite directions
We all seemed to find
My brother, the lost one
We all would divide

STRAIGHT JACKET

3,000 miles away
My mother with me
On that very sad day
My father was there
The police did arrive
My brother, my brother
So sad inside
He screamed,
Help me dad
I'll be good
His illness unwavering
His entire being
It never should
Have evolved to nothing
Existence in dictionary
No way to describe
The hell for my brother
Yet he still does survive.

TAKE ME AWAY

I grasped at love
First time bad
Second time worse
Insecure
Desperate
A great need of thirst
Take me away
From this sadness PLEASE
I often got on bended-knee
Asking for forgiveness
They were evil and cruel
Take me away
But I didn't want to go home

THE APARTMENT

The apartment is bare
No furniture
Little food
Your dog no longer there
The apartment
Empty, with pill bottles
The apartment
Social worker
Checking in and out
Doesn't change a thing
There will be always be doubt
Are you safe?
Are you fed?
Are you clean?
Do you ache?
Your illness is
Nothing that can be fixed
Until your end
And God will take you
Around the bend
And ease your pain
And change your being
To hopeful, safe,
Nothing in between

THE CELL PHONE

Does the phone speak to me?
How does it work?
I don't know my brother
It's just a perk
How can I see this? He asked over and over again
What have I missed
In my lifetime and present
This crazy technology
I never saw anything like this before
People can see me
Even walk out the door?
Like living in a time warp
You were cheated so much
Companion to love you
And call every day
An iPhone for you would
Truly pave the way
Things we take for granted
Amaze you as such
Your heart is pure
And ever so deep
Your track phone for now
Will keep us in touch
You are my brother
I love you baby so much

THE CLOSET

Like a lion's roar
Heard outside the door
To the closet escaped
And shivered with fear
Begged him to stop
He just couldn't hear
The rage in his voice
The screams in his throat
The fear they both felt
Exhaustion saved him
And then her
Afterwards it was a blur

DISTANCE

The distance is good
So far away
In miles that is
To protect me today
My heart still feels sadness
And yours so much worse
Your illness took over
It's simply a curse
The miles are long
But still don't prevent
The tears in our eyes
Of times in youth spent
You are my brother
And if truth is real
We will meet again
On other terms
And it will be your time
To feel good thoughts
And plan for your future

THE EDGE

Grasping, digging
Hanging on
To the side of a mountain
Yet not that strong
Labored breathing
Another dimension
Without well-being

THE INHERITANCE

My mother died first
My father then followed
The money was managed by two
Too much to swallow
Mistrust, Distrust!
Trying to section it to last longer
I need a TV
I have a bill
Not everyone had your best interest still
Of someone that's ill
We hear about it always
Down to the last $5,000
I sent it in one lump sum
The stress was too great
It did not make you well
It did not make you one
The money didn't last
That's all in the past

WHAT IS YOUR DAY?

Do you wake up and smile
Do you feel sad?
Sleep on the couch
Do you walk to the bathroom
No car makes it hard
Will your laundry be clean?
What are your thoughts?
Do you dream of a girl?
New York City
Do you wear the same clothes?
Do you sleep with your hoodie?
Do you cover yourself
Do you have a pillow
To relax your head
Slippers next to your makeshift bed
Can you grab a snack from your floor
So many empty wrappers
Do you take a walk
Down the same street
Do you have hope
While traveling
Your broken feet
What kind of day are you having?

THE KITCHEN

The scent of spaghetti
Made by my father
He tried so hard
To mentor and honor
Our family
Though broken
He would often crack jokes
And I would say
Dad – stop!
I'm embarrassed
Is this just a hoax?
My mom sometimes there
Brother the same
Smiles and frowns identical
The stare from empty eyes
They would turn into disturbed
Not his fault
The way he was created
The illness, the family,
Or un-family more often than not
To be seated at the tiny table for two
In the red kitchen
I often felt mostly blue

THE SCHOOL BUS

The day my brother traveled on a bus
A school bus for children with Downs Syndrome
Yet, that was not him
Curled in a corner
Like brick and mortar
Mental illness to them was all the same
The damage became much greater
The system labeled all insane

LET'S CLEAN THE HOUSE AND WE WILL BE LOVED

I'll fill the bucket
You grab the mop
I'll scrub each step
On the staircase
Towards her bed
And make it shine
Please just a moment
Do not cry or whine
Let's make toast
And bring hot tea
A loving note
From you and me
To mommy's bed
She will feel like a princess
And love us more
I was a little girl
And you a little boy
We did good together
Creating love
Cleaning the floor
And then when asked
We'd close the door

THE SOUL

Is there a soul?
In a deep dark hole?
Does it
Live with us after?
Why can't it speak?
It's buried too long
And way too deep
The soul should follow our every move
While living
And moving
The soul
Is part
Of our being
Although
We believe
Without even seeing
I'm praying my soul
Will speak to me
To help my brother
See there's another
Piece that will
Fill the puzzle
And create a heart
That's not broken

"Be involved again and again or they may be forgotten."

Francine Fuentes

THE WOMB

Inside and hidden
Safe and sound
Or, so we think
Then born is a human
Different than most
Voices speak to the baby
As if there's a host
Doctors can't fix it
No one can
In the womb
The beginning of man
Yet the brain
Is broken
It sees what's not there
Or maybe it is
We never dare
To ask the question
Or state it's not true
The newborn grows
Up and knows what it knows
And what it's told to do
No argument
Fixes
Inside the womb
And yet
Once the baby is born
The net is gone
And he is doomed
From then and now on

"They said I couldn't, but I did! "

Francine Fuentes

"They said I was stupid, they said to give up! Glad I didn't listen."

Francine Fuentes

IT'S ABOUT WHO WE CAN BECOME

What I'm told is what I am
Is who I am from outer space
Is who I am the human race
Is what I'm told how I began
Does future hold
What can I be?
They can't take that away from me
To Become what my future holds
I tell you now
That I behold
The key to strength
And trudging on
What I become is
More than they could know
It's more than math
Trigonometry
It's me plus 1
What I will be
Doubt what the critics say
I possess secrets that
May delay
The finished product
Is who I am
For doubting the voice
I am a Man

TREAT ME BADLY

Treat me badly
I deserved all of the abuse
It stemmed from many things

Treat me badly
I knew then I was loved
God seemed so far away

Treat me badly
Treat me badly
And I will stay, more than gladly
I will attempt to stay
In my brother's life

TWO FACED

Not in the normal sense
A face that changes
Throughout the day
From smiling
Laughing
And
Saying hello
To
What are you doing?
What have you done?
Leave me alone!
I can't help myself
My thoughts
Come and Go
There are bugs in the air
The TV talks to me
You were there
You know it's the truth
With the flow of cross arrows
I pray you'll regroup
Is that all that matters?

VENOM

The snake can sense
When to attack
They sliver slowly
Then pull back
The Strike, the strike
Their desire
The pain will feel
Like blazing fire
Humans stay on high alert
As snakes come in many forms
And varieties of dirt
Some sliver
Some Creep
Some stand tall
Some adorn
In hidden ways
On alert
Mental illness
Seems to stay
Can we trust a snake that hides
Can my brother believe the lies?

WATER

I can't wash myself
You don't understand
I can't describe
The feelings I have
It's been a year
Since I have bathed
I'll shower soon

"We all have it, to varying degrees – a piece of the mind that's different, creative to a fault-call it what you want; insanity, depression, mania, neurosis, phobia, lunacy, delusional, tormented, lost."

Francine Fuentes

WHAT DO YOU WANT TO BE WHEN YOU GROW UP?

Loved
A mother
A wife
Loved
A mother
A wife
Loved
A mother
A wife
Loved
A mother
A wife
LOVED

WHEN WILL YOU COME BACK?

When will you come back?
I promise I will
But right now I can't
I know you don't believe me
Or anyone at all
But you are loved
Please hold on

WHERE ARE YOU?

Each day I call your number
Sometimes twice or more
I know...
You don't ignore me
Your heart is way too pure
Something has upset you
Perhaps I try too hard
My mind is doing craziness
I don't mean to alarm

MOMMY IN LA

Mostly, I saw you once a year
You came to California
You were a breath of fresh air
What I loved most was
Sitting on my sofa
Holding your hand
Talking for hours
About your dreams
For me to move on to
A new life
And how difficult yours was
I wanted you to have more happy moments
And feel the ocean breeze
In Torrance, California
I wanted to please
I know you loved me with all your heart
And sometimes I fell off the chart
We are a product of our past
My memories of you
Have all come back
You loved me mommy
And I still love you

WHOSE LIFE?

The queasy feeling in my lower gut
The time I felt an entire knot
The blanket pulled above my head
Can't hide the demons outside my bed
A misfit I was
And forever will be
My brother afar is inside of me
I only was valued
When I fixed all the bugs
When thinking outside of them
My heart was then robbed
Of childhood dreams
I was the mother
Of a very sick boy
I was the child
Where was my joy?
Was it fair
Why my role?

WHY CAN'T I REMEMBER?

I try to relive
The baby boy
Who was a snuggly bundle of innocent joy
Why can't I remember?
You crawling around
I try and try
And there is no sound
Did I hold you?
Did I tell you
What you might be?
When you were young
Did you climb a tree?
I remember school days
Protecting you then
But want to go back to before it began
When your life was simple and we didn't know
Schizophrenia
Why did it have to be you?

MY BROTHER, THE WRITER

His mind not clear
He writes the facts
What's inside
What he lacks
Brilliant words
He tells the truth
What he's told
He knows how
The fog sets in
He drops his pen
Says he can't
The meds prevent
His truthful rant

WHY TRY?

When failing is easy
Test taking
Complete
60 seconds or less
Why bother
I'm just a mess
Concentrate, concentrate
Squeeze the brain
The vessels contract
Until heart bleeds remain
Learning is hard
With critical needs
Come up with a pill
To satisfy needs
The system
Requires
For those
That don't get it
It takes a long while
I wish to forget it

SHE WILL LEAVE ME!

If you marry him
If you move out
If you move in
Take your brother
Help with the baby

CONFORM

Stay here forever
You don't have to leave
Everything you need
Is here in this house
I must get out
I need to stretch my mind
I don't need a house
I need a home
I feel alone
Someone will love me
Someday they will
I'm not yet a mother
My brother is my sibling still
He can come to visit
But then he must go home
You try to take the easy road
By keeping ME at home

WINTER BOOTS

Traveling to the movie theatre
Wearing my brothers baby boots
Covered half of my feet
As I sludged through the snow
And did not feel the warmth
The back of my feet were full of snowflakes
By the time we arrived
Frostbite could have set in
My brother in shoes with holes
In a cold Philly winter
What the heck,
Why weren't we dressed?
From the elements
Poor, I guess

WORN OUT CLOTHES—-

Body Image
Fitting in
I would erase
The pain I felt
Of my disgrace
Frayed clothes
Missing buttons
Torn hose
Other girls
Adorned with style
I often wished
It was a trial
My counselor said
This is not ok
Your daughter needs clean clothes
Not tomorrow
TODAY!

"The truth is, no one took care of my brother."

Francine Fuentes

"Saying goodbye also means I no longer have that sick knot in my stomach."

Francine Fuentes

Chapter 3
The journey - the beginning? The end? Dysfunction !

There is so much more to my story to be included in my book but I believe I have buried the pain so I have written what I recollect, what stood out and what I wish could be a re-do.

I was born in Philadelphia and moved to California in my 20s. I drove away from an unhappy home while I was in an unhappy and abusive marriage to California. I left one set of problems and traveled to another. There was never encouragement to have my own thoughts, opinions and to be someone on my terms.

After I settled in California, I would travel to Philly to visit my parents. I would sleep on the floor as close as possible to the front door. It made me feel like I had control. In my mind, that was my safety net. I would be able to exit and return to MY home when I chose to. If I were in the bedroom in the back of the house it felt as if I were a prisoner.

The living room was cold and damp so I would keep an electric heater close to my body. My father was worried that my blanket would catch on fire and I was worried that I would never be able to leave their house.

I never told my parents the feelings I had of being trapped. My mom would make the bed comfortable for me. I felt guilty and sorry for my parents but I was sick and tired of being responsible for everyone's well being! Always begging for love! I was pretty messed up!

When morning would come, I would feel better about visiting because I was one day closer to leaving their house.
The day my mother was diagnosed with cancer was shattering. My mom fell apart after receiving the devastating news. She was 60 years old. Doctors are only human, I told her. They don't know everything! I believe it was three months after diagnosis that she died.

I flew to Philly the morning I received the call from my father that my mother was on her deathbed. She passed away a half hour before I got there. I remember going into the hospital room. It was dark. Her hair was totally white. She was a vibrant redhead until she became ill with cancer. On the way to Philadelphia, I sat next to a couple on the plane and began talking about my mom. They were involved with some sort of spiritual group and I guess the timing was right. They suggested I take a lit candle into my mom's hospital room and pray. I talked to her but I'm not sure she heard me. I asked her to let me know she was ok at her final destination. I promised I would care for Ronnie. Promises?

I believe she wanted the best for me. I wanted the best for her! I wanted my mom to take some of my burden. My mom was born in England. During war time she and her sister were sent to live in an orphanage as their mother (my grandmother) had to work. Their little sister stayed home. I can only imagine how sad and insecure she was during those days. I can only imagine what I would have been had my mother left me. Stronger?

I wish I would have met my grandmother from my mother's side. I wish my grandmother would have been able to travel to America. That was the plan. She too died from cancer. My brother would have had more family. If everything had been normal.

WHERE DID YOU GO?

Sometimes my mom would go to the hospital for a procedure. I was young so I don't remember what it was for, but I do remember I would cry to our neighbor and she would reassure me that my mother would return. There were several procedures that followed. My mom would be gone for days at a time. I was always anxious that she wouldn't come home. I didn't want to be the mother. I didn't want to be alone. I didn't want to be abandoned.

FIX MY FAMILY

My mom and I were close but she had strong opinions about many things. The best for me would have been to eliminate the feelings of constant guilt! The best for me would have been to be a child that wasn't responsible for everyone's happiness. I couldn't fix my parents! I couldn't fix myself. I wouldn't feel abandonment, loneliness and emptiness if I would have just died. That was always my out! I had the choice to not feel pain if it got too bad. That's what kept me going for many years. Options!

My mother and father asked me to travel to England with them and I was always afraid to leave my home (nothing behind). I never went because if I were out of sight, I'd be forgotten.

THE INVISIBLE MAN

The invisible man would make things better for my mother. I was told he was a family friend. He often took care of things. I liked him at first and then as I grew older, it turned to dislike, distrust and just being pissed off! I remember at one point telling him to stay away. He called me to say don't marry your first husband. It will destroy your mother. I told him to mind his own business. I thought he was successful when in reality he was just an old man of 60! Well, I was younger then. Why was he telling me what to do???

LUNCH IN PHILLY

I loved when my mom would meet me at my work place in Philadelphia to have lunch with me. There was a fresh salad bar down some side street that we would go to and it was the most delicious salad. I loved those times. I think she was proud of me when I would be dressed in my suit and high heels. I felt like the girl on the TV show *That Girl*. I wanted it to be my time. I created a fairytale for myself when working in the city.

MY FATHER

I don't remember a whole lot about my father growing up
except that he worked a lot. He tried to comfort me when
a boyfriend broke up with me. I thought I was going to die.
In reality, had he stayed with me I probably would have. My
boyfriend's mother told us that we had to get married and I
recall my father telling me if you marry him, mommy will
leave me. I didn't marry him. Thank God. But why would
my mother leave my father because of something I did? I
remember my friend's father and I always felt they cared more
about their daughters because they seemed stronger. He was
strong but not at expressing himself with me.

I REMEMBER

My father, the holster, a ring, cans full of coins, the attic with his hidden treasures! Tools in the shed, bikes with no frames, signs with no names, breakfast trays by the dozen, nuts, bolts, silver spoons and a heated floor in the kitchen.

I'M TOLD

I'm told my father's sister had Down's Syndrome and that she was sent to an institution.. I guess this happened often back then. I never met her but saw photographs. Those that were different, forgotten, thrown away, much like now! Is it getting better? Are differences being accepted? I hope it improves.

LIGHTEN UP

Have a drink., Nah, I don't like that stuff. Why? Just be dad!
Relax! Show me you are my father.

HEAVINESS

Dark curtains in the living room, yet not much living. Heavy curtains, my father sewed them, he knew how. The light was well hidden, not sure why. God made windows to let the light in. I rarely felt light-hearted!

The Bust, the porcelain bust in a corner of the living room. Beautiful yet scary! More eerie than anything. My mother saved pennies to buy her stuff! My mom loved to host dinner get-togethers. I wish I would have attended more of them. I was too busy escaping! Not sure where I escaped to. My head was always in the same lonely place. I remember the sofa that had an odd shape that was not built for comfort with plastic covers. The plastic would stick to my legs. Not a cozy home.

TRIED TO ESCAPE BY MARRYING THE WRONG GUY -- 1ST MARRIAGE

Before I married the second guy, my father said to me, "If you marry him, mommy will leave me!" Why was I responsible for their marriage? So much like the abuse with the previous boyfriend. This guy never worked, would beat and berate me. He was anti Semitic. A miserable 16 years. It was f'd... up! I finally left! Actually I didn't leave anything. There was no security, no love, no partnership and no man!!

MY HUSBAND

Finally, I met yet another guy who became my husband for the past 32 years and he actually goes to work every day. He loves and cares for me. He has never hit me and is an extremely gentle man. I won the lottery. The sad part is that my mother never met him. I remember telling my mother about him and she said she was happy for me. That conversation took place when she was on her deathbed.

PICTURE PERFECT

For the first few years of my marriage, I would go to sleep with makeup on so that my husband would not see the real me. I didn't like what I saw. I was desperately trying to hold on to his love. In my mind, the real me would not have been enough. More craziness!

I was always fearful of having a child. I guess from my history. I finally met someone that showed me I could be a mommy. We have one amazing son together. I like to think he would have been the bright light for my mother.

HOMEWORK

As a child, I wanted someone to sit with me and help me with my homework. I used to carry books all of the time and play librarian to make me look smart. I must have done some homework, but I don't remember.

PAMPERED

When my mother would visit me, she could breathe. The goal was to ease her pain. The dress shop in Hermosa Beach, California was a happy place for my mom and me. I wanted to spoil her. Pleasing her made me happy. She would pick out a piece of clothing and I would put it on layaway for her and then mail it to her home on pay day. I could make her happy... for a short time. She had a break from the turmoil at her home.

DARK SECRETS

Every family has the shadow of darkness. Even *Leave it to Beaver* families. Manipulation, silent treatment often came into play. Guilt was an everyday feeling in my face.

My father visited my sister in California and then came to Colorado to visit me. He passed away while in Colorado. Before my parents died, they helped my brother move into his own apartment (subsidized housing). He has been there for close to 40 years and still lives there today. I'm not sure how he has managed. Maybe the voices also tell him how to survive. He Might Be Schizophrenic, But he is NOT crazy!

DEATH

Headstones together. Funny how you can be buried side-by-side but separate when living. A gravesite is a place for others to visit.
My Brother was now alone!

ABOUT THE AUTHOR

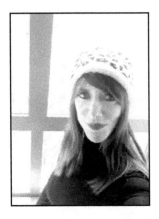

Francine Fuentes is drawn to helping those that struggle. Being told she was not capable of success from a very young age, she weaved a pattern of her own, showing others that they can learn, dream and be successful! In turn, it opened up out of the ordinary and extraordinary opportunities for her.

Francine earned a certificate in Business Entrepreneurship which helped shape her desire to write her first book. She has presented numerous times at colleges throughout the state of Florida on the subject of judgment, labeling and making a difference in others' lives.

She was born in Philadelphia and currently resides in Clearwater, Florida. Married to Al and mother of son, Gabriel, she learned quickly that she did not have most of the answers although she experienced many of the lessons. Francine's brother had a lesson for her, and that is to always notice the mentally ill and the homeless. They were born to someone. They deserve life. She knows we all experiment looking for the perfect life and that what we think the end product could be truly open doors for the unexpected.

Move forward! Only look back when you want to be reminded of the direction you are not following! Mental illness shaped her world.